Face Lifting (Latest findings)

- Face and throat muscle-toning exercises
- Nutritional dietary supplements
- Top 10 Anti-Aging tips

by Marie van Huellen

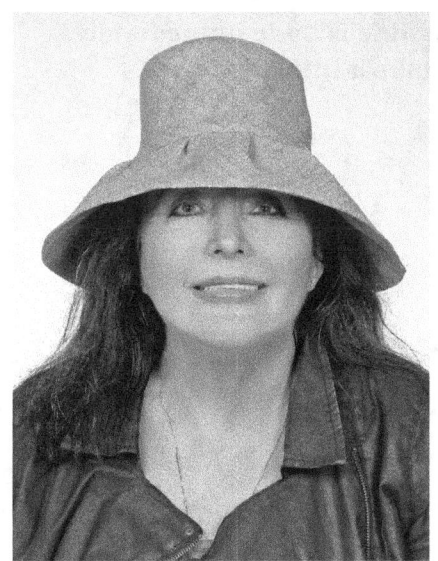

Growing older without aging …

or:

**"The impossible is done immediately,
 miracles take a little longer!"**

Index

- The three pillars

Foreword

When we encounter a person, we look them in the eyes, we look at their face. The face conveys the first impression we have of a person. Then we look at their hands and their figure. It does not matter to us whether the face is beautiful or not. What appeals to us is its expression, its harmony, that it is cared for, what it radiates.

Your face is your business card!

Every person is subject to the natural aging process, which cannot be stopped but it can certainly be slowed. Starting at age 25, the cells in our body lose their regenerative ability. They are no longer able to store enough oxygen. The aging process sets in.

What can we 'do' to ensure that our face and throat do not 'age' as we grow older? When we exercise our body, the muscles underneath the skin are firmed up, toned and tightened. The same applies to our facial muscles. We shall exercise the muscles beneath our skin and achieve an outstanding result : 'Firm facial features'.

The skin is the largest organ of our body.

It conceals our musculature. According to the dictionary, 'muscles serve to move the body, the organs and the face'. They are contractile, meaning, they are made up of tissue that is contractable. That is our starting point. We shall exercise the muscles of our face. Two, three minutes per day, six times a week, are required in order to achieve a great result.

Selected dietary supplements, specifically tailored to nourish the skin, together with a good skin care routine, round off our beauty program perfectly. The result is sensational :
We do not age as we grow older.

The skin

The skin is the outer covering of our body, our largest sensory organ. Over the years, it becomes increasingly **dryer**, **thinner** and **loses its elasticity**. Due to significant hormonal changes in our body - especially after menopause - perspiration and sebaceous glands, responsible for suppleness and moisturising the skin, are less active and the skin **dries out**. The sun, indoor heating, pollution, poor nutrition, smoking and alcohol all contribute in speeding up the aging process of the skin.

Gradually the fat cells under the epidermis disappear, collagen formation (a structural substance) decreases, hyaluronic acid (skin moisture) is minimized, the skin becomes **thinner**. The skin aging process can be compared to that of an apple which shrinks as it ages due to decreased moisture content. The skin loses its elasticity, wrinkles appear.

Regular physical exercise keeps a body in shape, it retains its youthful form. The same applies to our face. Muscles that are not exercised become **limp** like the muscles in our face. This is where we begin – we shall exercise our face and our throat here.

If we want to successfully prevent the formation of wrinkles, then the best time for that is now – take the opportunity here to achieve maximum success with minimal effort.

A skin cell

It is made up of:

- Epidermis (outer skin)
- Dermis (corium)
- Subutaneous tissue (hypodermis)

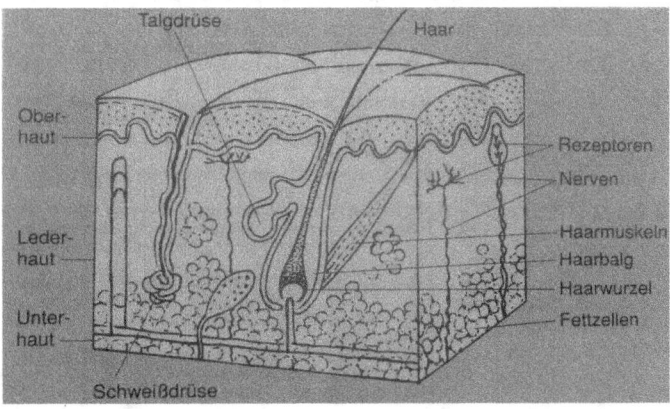

According to Pschyrembel, the skin is: "The largest human organ, covering the entire body (1.62 square metres), rich in water, proteins, lipids (fats), low in carbohydrates and contains electrolytes."

The musculature

Face muscles exercises – also called 'isometric exercises' – condition the muscles underneath the face.

By definition, a muscle is a fleshy part of the body that produces physical movement by alternatively contracting and relaxing.

It has been scientifically proven that a muscle has to be exercised for at least six seconds every day for it to retain its tensioning ability and not become limp (isometric exercises).
'Isometric' is the definition of the voltage change produced in the muscle at a constant tension (contraction time). As described below, we create a tension field on our skin to carry out the exercises.

Facial muscles

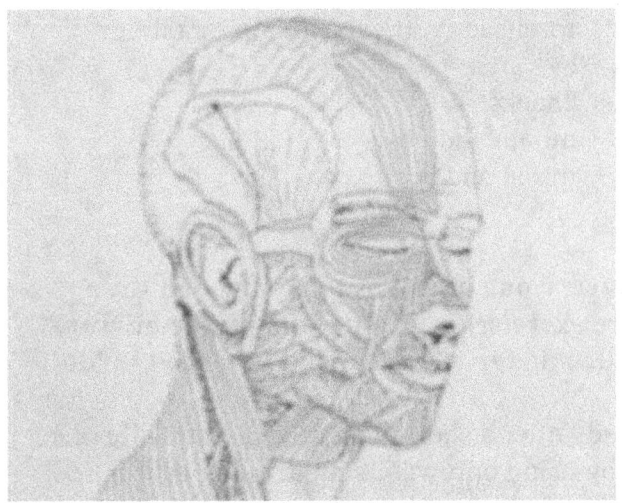

We commence here and skillfully exercise the musculature beneath the skin. We push and pull (force and counter force) (as shown in the photographic illustrations) using our fingers and produce a tension field that is held for six seconds.

Then we gently relax, we finish the exercise, we let go. Exercise by exercise, we improve.
We are exercising the:

- forehead (vertical and horizontal lines)
- eye area
- cheeks
- mouth and nose
- throat and neck

Not every one of us has to go through the entire exercise program. Look in the mirror and decide for yourself what you need to 'do'!

Already after a short practice run, you will notice that by using only very simple methods it is possible to firm up facial features. Doing the facial muscle exercises will become a pleasant routine. Be careful you don't become addicted!

The first step is the hardest – or maybe not?!

We sit down at a table, place a mirror in front of us and commence the exercises. At the beginning, we place our elbows on the table for support and make a start, depending on the exercise and which facial area we want to work on.

Over time, as the exercises have become second nature to us, we'll no longer need the table. We practice at night in bed, in the morning, at noon, while travelling in a plane, in a train, whenever we feel like it. For best results, six times a week. And when no one is watching, because initially 'pulling a face' is unavoidable, as is a 'funny face' - a stranger may misunderstand exactly what it is you are doing.

And be prepared for your fellow citizens: "Mrs Soandso, when are you ever going to grow old...?" May happen!

Effort is rewarded and the result will be outstandingly unique: 'Growing older without aging!'

The exercises are not as difficult as they may sound to some. Look at it this way: "Nothing is eaten as hot as it is prepared!"

I. The exercises
(Isometric facial muscle-toning
exercises)

1. Exercise
Wide smile

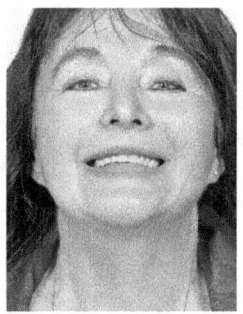

To become aware of our facial muscles, we break into a wide smile and are 'consciously' aware of all the muscles in our face.

Notes

2. Exercise

Forehead – vertical lines

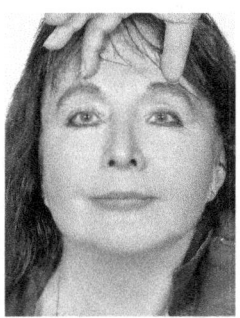

To work on vertical forehead lines, we place both index fingers firmly in the middle of each eyebrow and gently pull the eyebrows to either side of our face. **At the same time**, we contract the muscle between the eyebrows into a frown. Push/pull, we produce the tension field. Maximum tension, hold for six seconds. Slowly relax.

Frown lines don't stand a chance!

Notes

3. Exercise – also a concluding exercise (basic exercise)
Forehead – horizontal lines

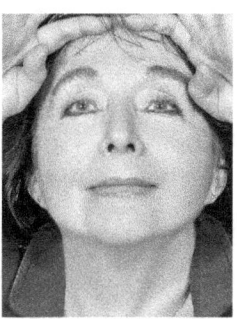

To work on horizontal forehead lines, we place both index fingers firmly at the top of the forehead, pulling gently upwards with each finger and **at the same time** tensing our forehead muscles down towards our nose. We create a tension field. Maximum tension, hold for six seconds. Slowly relax.

Please note!
This exercise not only works against horizontal forehead lines but should also be used **after** every exercise session! It restores proper muscle positioning and shape.

Notes

4. Exercise

Eye area

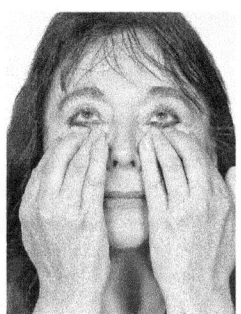

To perform this exercise, we place our elbows on the table and the fingertips of either hand gently below each eye, while **at the same time** tensing our eye muscles to move upwards. Maximum tension, hold for six seconds. Slowly relax. This exercise tightens the eye area below each eye and reduces the appearance of tear bags.

Notes

5. Exercise - Cheeks
(basic exercise)
- **Plumps up cheeks and face for a youthful appearance**

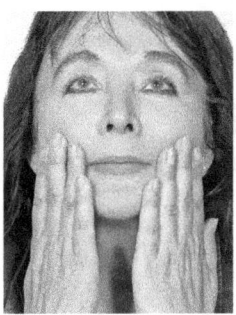

We rest on our elbows, place the four fingers of each hand together flat on each cheek and push upwards while **at the same time** opening our mouth and using the muscles around our nose to pull downwards to produce the tension field. Maximum tension, hold for six seconds. Slowly relax.

Notes

6. Exercise
Throat - front
(basic exercise)

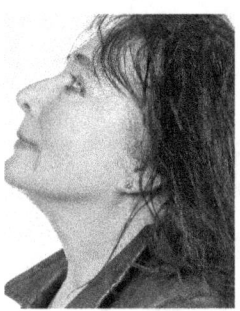

To exercise the front part of our throat, we sit up straight on a chair, tilt our head back as far as it will go, pull our lower lip up over our upper lip and pull up the entire front throat area with that movement as hard as we can. Maximum tension, hold for six seconds. Slowly relax.

Notes

Exercise for the lateral throat area

Either side of the throat, the right and the left, are exercised as follows:

Left side:

We take our left hand, place the palm against our left ear, push gently upwards and **at the same time** using the muscles of our left cheek, pull down. Maximum tension, hold for six seconds.

Right side:

We take our right hand, place the palm against our right ear, push gently upwards and **at the same time** using the muscles of our right cheek, pull down. Maximum tension, hold for six seconds.

Notes

7. Exercise

Nose area

This exercise prevents the shapely nose of our youth from becoming an increasingly elongated 'structure' because nose and ears increase in size as we grow older.

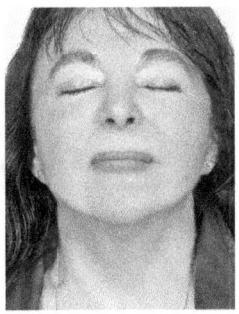

We concentrate on our nose, the tip of our nose and, using the inner nose muscles, reach the nose stem, located between our eyebrows. Maximum tension, hold for six seconds.

For the Buddhists among us, this is also an exercise to find the third eye, which improves our understanding, insight and awareness!

Notes

8. Exercise

Mouth area

For our lips to retain their natural full shape and form, we place a finger firmly on either side of our mouth (right and left), pulling outwards, creating a tension field as we purse our lips and pull our muscles inwards. Push/pull, maximum tension, hold for six seconds.

Drooping mouth corners don't stand a chance here!

Notes

Note

Not every one of us has to go through the entire program of eight exercises. As a rule, the three basic exercises suffice: exercise no. 3, no. 5 and no. 6. Hard to believe but just three exercises per day (two/three minutes) and we've succeeded in tricking age.
In addition it is important to take two key dietary supplements: collagen lift drink and hyaluronic acid capsules (only recently released on the market) – both strengthen the skin from the inside. Collagen is the substance that resurrects the collagen fibres (scaffolding) of the skin and hyaluronic acid acts against the skin drying out. And it benefits all of your skin, not only the face and throat.

The result:

'A sensational result. Growing older without aging!'

The mirror shall decide where 'it's needed'.

To clarify:

The facial muscle-toning exercises are based on a method called 'isometric', meaning: by using our fingers, we create a tension field. Force and counter force, maximum tension, hold for six seconds. Gentle strength is wanted, no hard jolting or tearing in any one direction. Ideally six times a week, wherever possible, at home, in bed, in the train, on a plane, whenever we feel like it.
And the result? "Fantastic!"

Facial expressions

Over time we develop an eye for how woefully most of us treat our face. At every suitable or unsuitable opportunity, we put a frown on our forehead, furrow our face deep in thought and push half our face to the heavens using our palm, resting on our elbows … In a young face, this may all still appear quite cute and charming, yet over time deep permanent lines and wrinkles will establish themselves in our face. Lines which can no longer be erased. That is why, and because it is an easy thing to do, everyone should pay attention to their habits, observe themselves, and acquire gentle facial mimicry, ideally a pokerface …

Mimicry is defined as: "The ability to convey mood or feelings in support of verbal expression, using not only our face but also body postures and hand gestures."

II. Nutritional dietary supplements
(available in shops)

1) Collagen

2) Hyaluronic acid

1) Collagen

Collagen is a protein, critical in the skin's regenerative structure and elasticity. It is responsible for maintaining supple, wrinkle-free skin. Clinical trials of women aged 33 – 59 have shown that just 10 g of collagen peptide ingested daily produced a significant reduction in small wrinkles after 12 weeks, as opposed to the group of women receiving a placebo. Deep wrinkles were softened, skin thickness increased, as well as skin moisture levels.

What is Beauty Collagen?
Beauty Collagen is a natural product, consisting of 97% type I collagen. This is exactly the type of protein that is essential for the structure and elasticity of the skin.
Beauty Collagen stimulates the body's own collagen production in the skin cells, producing a visible improvement in skin texture after only a few weeks. The skin holds more moisture, appears smoother, fresh, and wrinkles seem to lose their depth.

Beauty Collagen -
- ensures tighter, more supple skin
- reduces fine lines and wrinkles
- has clinically proven effectiveness
- promotes collagen production in the skin
- increases moisture retention in the skin
- has high bio-availability
- is an all natural product
(available in shops as **Collagen-Lift-Drink**)

(Source: www.vitaminexpress.org/beauty-collagen)

2) Hyaluronic acid

What is hyaluronic acid?

Hyaluronic acid is a natural product. Its name is derived from the Greek - 'hyalos' meaning 'glassy', and it is found throughout the body, with 50% of it in the skin, in the spaces between the cells of the dermis. The gelatinous substance is produced by stromal cells, plumping up the skin, supporting collagen and elastin fibres and scavenging free radicals. Unfortunately, this effect does not last. Already from age 25 onwards these deposits start to empty bit by bit. Gradually, the skin stops producing collagen. Elasticity decreases, and from age 40 the skin stores less moisture, deeper wrinkles can begin to form. Finally at age 60 then, it may be that only 10% of it is left in the person's body. To compensate for the lack of this precious beauty substance, **hyaluronic acid** is available commercially in both **capsule** form and as a **gel**. Hyaluronic acid is an all natural product and has high bio-availability.

(Source: 'Natura Vitalis')

Note:

As we can see, due to scientific findings it is possible for us today to care for the skin externally using cosmetics, as well as to also regenerate it from the inside using nutrition. Add to that our isometric facial muscle-toning exercises and we will achieve a sensational result which will not be surpassed.

Can we stop wrinkles through nutrition?

According to one US study, we can.

The more vitamin C (collagen formation), the fewer wrinkles is the motto. Large amounts of this beauty vitamin are found in the kiwi fruit, berries, red capsicum, cabbages and, of course, vitamin C tablets. Vitamin C is water-soluble and the body simply expels excess amounts. As well as being good for the skin, vitamin C also maintains good overall health.

Olive oil is worth mentioning because of its unsaturated fatty acids. They provide the skin with improved elasticity and resilience. Or take one capsule of fish oil daily.

The least expensive anti-aging substance is water. One glass. Already 10 minutes after enjoying a glass of water our skin is has a better supply of blood and oxygen. The famous '2 litres a day' will do it!

Exercise is everything. It improves the flow of blood and nutrients to the skin.

Conclusion:

Getting older? Not now!

Skin care

The cosmetics industry offers plenty of products that we are supposed to buy – from deep pore cleansing scrubs to peelings and an infinitely wide range of creams, masks and booster vials. Whether all of this is of use in the end and benefits anyone other than the beauty industrialists, remains to be seen. Experience has shown that unless you happen to work in a mine underground, daily cleansing of the face, throat and décolleté using only lukewarm water and rinsing with cold water (be careful - rosacea) is enough. A daily, 24 hour moisturising cream, free of mineral oils and parabeens and for special occasions a moisturising mask or booster vial – that should be all. Optimal skin care is a moisturizing day cream and a regenerating night cream in one 'pot', containing phytohormones, vitamins and nourishing oils. Depending on your age and skin type.

It is not for this **'guide'** to list skin care tips. That topic has been reported on since Adam and Eva, and that Cleopatra bathed in milk is known throughout the whole world!

Internationally famous!
(Hollywood, too, is practicing)

The famous **'workouts'** - classic facial muscle-
toning exercises!

        Victoria Beckham (38)
        Julia Roberts (45)
        Susan Sarandon (66)

They all do them.

And last but not least, that special beauty mark:

    'My beautiful flaw! '

Have fun and keep up the good work!

III. Top 10 Anti-Aging Tips

1) **Brain training**
2) **Healthy diet**
3) **Antioxidants**
4) **Eat a little less every day**
5) **Oral hygiene**
6) **Meditation**
7) **8 hours sleep**
8) **Sports**
9) **Breathing exercises**
10) **Hormones**

Addresses:

Deutsche Gesellschaft für Anti-Aging-Medizin (GSAAM)
Josephspitalstrasse 15
80331 Munich / Germany
Tel.: +49 (0)89/7435-7890
www.gesam.de

Europäische Vereinigung für
Aktives Anti-Aging e.V. (EVAA)
Karl-Heine-Strasse 99
04229 Leipzig / Germany
Tel.: +49 (0)341/491251

SAABA Swiss Austrian Association for
Better Aging
Dr.med.Christoph Winkler
Spital Oberengadin
7503 Samedan / Switzerland
Fax: +41(0)818525310

Institute of Biomedical Aging Research of
The Austrian Academy of Sciences
Dr. Ignaz-Seipel-Platz 2
1010 Vienna / Austria

The World Anti-Aging Academy of Medicine
The First Global Entity in Anti-Aging and
Regenerative Medicine
Medicine -

www.ingramcontent.com/pod-product-compliance
Lightning Source LLC
Chambersburg PA
CBHW072251310526
45795CB00011B/916